Intermittent Fasting for Beginners

Which type fits into your lifestyle? Health benefits and much more

written by Flygirl

.

Content

No new trend

If you start to deal with the trends of nutrition/nutritional medicine, you will be flooded with nutritional methods, dietary supplements, ... when you do a detailed research.

As a completely normal person who wants to find a nutrition method for himself that integrates well into the individual's everyday life, this means researching for hours or even days.

Not only does your own research flood you with a wealth of information, but there are also friends or relatives with whom you might discuss the subject. This leads to the fact that still many further opinions rain down on you, experiences, which made friends with this or that nourishing method, ...

Not everything that works for others or fits in well with their everyday lives is also right and goal-oriented for you.

Everybody's everyday life is different!

Everyone's diet is different!

Everyone`s metabolism is different!

The jobs are different (office or construction site, ...).

Are you single or do you have a family with children?

Do I gain weight quickly or can I eat sweet food all day without gaining weight?

In addition, there is a flood of information on which diseases intermittent fasting can prevent or even positively influence their course.

But every person is different!

Intermittent fasting seems to be a new trend, but people are already practicing intermittent fasting, yes one can say, as long as humanity exists.

If we look at the history of mankind, one can clearly say: Intermittent fasting is actually the original form of human nutrition!

Thousands of years ago, not even 100 years ago, people were dependent on what nature had to offer them as food.

Regular meals were usually a no-no.

The food was heavily dependent on the place where one lived, the season, was it just a peaceful time or war, were harvests washed away shortly before bringing in, did rain masses, a drought destroyed everything that should bring one through the winter,

...

There were times when you didn't know if you had something to eat the next day, and if so, if it was enough to get you full.

Today we go into a supermarket and face an oversupply of food.

In all religions there are fasting rituals and therefore in most cultures there is a long tradition of fasting. The knowledge of the positive effect of fasting is therefore very old.

For a variety of reasons, the fasting was deliberately carried out:

➢ detoxification of the body
➢ unfold spiritual energies
➢ to purify the mind through meditation during lent

➤ ...

Conclusion: Fasting, especially intermittent fasting, is actually in our blood.
It is something that can still be found in human genetics today and therefore it is a completely natural way of fasting that has only been rediscovered.

What is intermittent fasting?

Intermitterre comes from the Latin and means interrupt.

Intermittent fasting is also called part-time fasting or interval fasting.

Interval fasting is a kind of "timetable" or "eating rhythm".

You benefit from the advantages of fasting, but without the stress and weakness of real hunger.

During intermittent fasting, everyone defines his or her time window in which food is supplied.

The nice thing are the different "timetables" from which you can choose.

Which of the possible fasting models is the right one for you depends on your individual circumstances, your daily routine, your family situations, ...

Intermittent fasting also helps to improve or realign the different processes in the body:

➢ Improve blood values
➢ Improve cholesterol levels

- ➤ accelerate your fat metabolism again
- ➤ to prevent diseases
- ➤ stimulate repair processes in the body
- ➤ Improve your stress resistance
- ➤ to get a nicer skin
- ➤ to feel happier again
- ➤ ...

Intermittent fasting is not a diet, rather it becomes a lifestyle after the transition phase.

Health benefits

Basically, there are hardly any medical studies on intermittent fasting that have a high scientific conclusiveness.

However, it has been proven that intermittent fasting is much easier for many people to maintain and is more sustainable than trying one diet after another. The introduction to intermittent fasting means a high degree of self-discipline and stamina.

However, if the chosen model is then integrated into everyday life and your body has become accustomed to the chosen rhythm, intermittent fasting is something of a "self-runner".

Which effects does interval fasting have on your body?

Body Weight

As you certainly know, the body can survive well without food for a long time.

It is also important during intermittent fasting: drinking, drinking, drinking, because without fluid the body very quickly gets problems.

Fluids in this case means as much water as possible!

And yes, there are so many opinions out there how much water you should drink during a day, ...

We have different weights, different genders, different ages, different jobs, live in different climates, ...

I personally like the information's I find on this site:

A look into history shows: People have often survived times when they had little or no access to food.

The difference between intermittent fasting and the many highly praised diets is easy to summarize: since your body has continuous fasting phases during intermittent fasting and food intake is healthy and balanced during the eating phases, you won't fall into the trap of the yo-yo effect, which often occurs with all diets.

The meal breaks during the fasting hours lead to the fact that your body nourishes itself from the body's own reserves.

The stored glycogen (liver and muscles) and fat reserves are "eaten up".

For the metabolism this means it learns to switch faster back and forth between carbohydrate burning and fat burning.

You get into a so-called "ketogenic metabolism":

From a certain point in time - especially if you eat a balanced and healthy diet and keep your carbohydrate intake as low as possible - your muscles and liver will no longer have enough glycogen to produce energy.

At this point, ketones are formed, which now produce energy from the body's own fat reserves. By reducing calories and changing to a ketogenic metabolism during intermittent fasting, it is possible to achieve a body fat reduction of up to 90 % over time.

➢ The ketogenic metabolism is possible without a Keto nutrition!

➢ Keto nutrition can be an addition to intermittent fasting (More information about Keto Nutrition for Beginners you find in my guide: Keto for Beginners)

90 % sounds like a lot, but when intermittent fasting is performed with great discipline and stamina over a long period of time, it is a proven value.

But you should always bear in mind that everybody is different, reaches the ketogenic metabolism at different speeds and then also reduces the body's own reserves in different ways.

For some people, the pounds fall quickly at the beginning and slowly afterwards.

Other people experience a continuous - but also slower - weight reduction.

Especially with these people, the following applies: don't give up, your body is just designed that way!

But the positive effects of weight loss can be seen in everyone: your mood gets better, you are less irritable, your self-esteem gets better again!

Metabolism

However, the limited information provided by scientific studies on the subject of intermittent fasting has led to this conclusion:

➢ Fats are reduced by the new flexibility of the fat metabolism and the ketogenic metabolism
➢ Your stress resistance improves
➢ Inflammatory processes in your body are regulated much earlier and better by your body itself

➢ Your insulin resistance is positively influenced (an even insulin release reduces hunger attacks)

Although there are only a very small number of conclusive scientific studies dealing with intermittent fasting, scientists and doctors have positive experiences from daily practice.

➢ <u>Blood</u>
the insulin levels in the blood improve - decrease

➢ <u>Liver</u>
increased insulin sensitivity in the liver can be detected

➢ <u>Bowel</u>
there is less inflammation in the intestine and energy absorption may be reduced

➢ <u>Muscle</u>
within the muscle there is an increased insulin sensitivity, less inflammation and as a result an increased effectiveness

➢ <u>Fat Cells</u>

the fat metabolism is changed very positively in some chemical processes, which supports fat reduction

➢ Heart

the resting pulse decreases, blood pressure is lowered and the resilience in stressful situations is improved

➢ Brain

The ability of the brain to withstand stress also increases in stressful situations. The cognitive functions improve and there are fewer signs of inflammation here as well

Aging process

When and how fast every human being ages is given to us by our genetics.

All the positive effects of intermittent fasting on your body will slow down your individual aging process.

It has been proven that fasting and the newly developed stress resistance, for example, protect the cells a lot better from any DNA damage.

The so-called risk markers for diabetes, cardiovascular diseases, ageing and even cancer are reduced.

Diabetes

As already mentioned, there are not yet many scientific studies on the positive effects of intermittent fasting in humans.

However, researchers at a university in California have tested the effect of intermittent fasting on overweight mice and mice with diabetes.

They used a 7:4 method: 7 days the mice could eat uncontrolled, then a fasting period of 4 days followed.

Already after a few months the mice were cured of their diabetes!

On the one hand, this had to do with weight loss during the fasting periods, but what was decisive was what happened in connection with the pancreas (produces insulin):

It is well known that diabetes is caused by an increased blood sugar level (excess glucose).

If we are healthy, insulin causes our cells to absorb glucose directly from the blood.

If one suffers from diabetes, the cells lose their sensitivity to insulin, which in turn means that the pancreas no longer produces insulin.

In the diabetes mice of the research study, the pancreas started producing insulin again. The pancreas was able to initiate repair mechanisms and stimulate cell regeneration.

Subsequently, it was observed that the pancreas decreased in size during the fasting period of 4 days and increased in size again during the 7-day eating period.

As a result of this change from smaller to larger, the pancreas has regenerated to such an extent that it has become a healthy and fully functional organ again.

This seems almost like a miracle and the leading researcher of this mouse study asked himself understandably whether intermittent fasting can have the same effects on people suffering from diabetes.

With a clinical examination and 100 overweight diabetes subjects, he then performed the following test:

An interval lasted 30 days. Within these 30 days, the subjects could eat without restriction for 25 days. The remaining 5 days the food supply was restricted according to a given plan.

After only 3 months (3 cycles) there were very big improvements in blood sugar levels and this without any side effects.

It is to be hoped that there will be real scientific and clinical studies on this subject in the future. Many people with diabetes could be helped in this way. Without taking the diabetes medication, which is burdened with many side effects, the body has the possibility to heal itself by intermittent fasting.

Cancer

A study at the University of Texas investigated the effect of intermittent fasting on leukemia.

Children suffer mainly from ALL (acute lymphoblastic leukemia).

Adults, on the other hand, usually suffer from AML (acute myeloid leukemia).

Only 15 % suffer from ALL.

In the case of ALL, the B and T cells of the white blood cells (immune defense) are affected.

In AML, the macrophages and granulocytes of the white blood cells are affected.

In both ALL and AML, these cells remain in an immature state and are therefore unable to perform the tasks assigned to them.

Through their uncontrolled proliferation, they displace the healthy cells until anemia and frequent infections occur.

And as it is usual with cancer, the diseased cells migrate into healthy tissue, where they cause further major problems.

How can intermittent fasting lead to the disappearance of cancer cells?

In tests on mice with ALL, intermittent fasting has completely inhibited cancer development.

The interval chosen for these tests was 1:2: eat 1 day, fast 1 day.

Already after 7 weeks! in most mice, the cancer cells had almost completely disappeared. The organs were healthy again and the small number of cancer cells still present behaved like active and healthy cells.

The mouse test group, which was still fed "normally", showed an increase in cancer cells.

One insight that unfortunately is not yet available is the long-term effect, or more precisely the question: Does intermittent fasting become ineffective when the cancer cells have become accustomed to the rhythm?

Further studies and tests are needed here!

However, intermittent fasting can be a possibility for people suffering from ALL and AML - especially at an early stage - to recover the diseased cells.

There are no side effects (like chemotherapy, ...) and it is certainly worth a try.

It will also be interesting to see whether the same or similar successes of cell regeneration can also be achieved with other types of cancer.

Neurodegenerative Diseases

Alzheimer's disease is the most common neurodegenerative disease worldwide and cannot be cured.

For this reason, it is important to look for ways to prevent the outbreak of the disease.

First studies show that intermittent fasting has the potential to prevent an outbreak or to reduce the severity of the progression.

In 9 out of 10 patients who tried intermittent fasting, there was a very strong improvement in Alzheimer's symptoms.

Studies of Huntington's and Parkinson's also suggest that intermittent fasting can protect against these diseases.

Brain

Autophagy plays a major role with increasing age, because it loses its ability to break down ineffective and old organelles (parts of the cell plasma) into their components and then rebuild new cells from these.
This leads to more and more cell damage.
This has a particular effect on the brain.
Alzheimer's, for example, is caused by a deposit of such plaques.

Through intermittent fasting, a cycle is stimulated again, so to speak:

- ➤ If the body receives less or no food, it falls back on other sources in the body.
- ➤ For energy generation these are all fat stores
- ➤ Amino acids are necessary for the production of proteins and other molecules
- ➤ Amino acids are broken down into proteins by autophagy
- ➤ The body first takes proteins that are older and no longer function efficiently
- ➤ The molecule waste in the cells is reduced and the proteins are renewed

Psyche

Why are you thinking about starting intermittent fasting?

You want to change your diet in the long run, eat healthier and more consciously!

You want to get your weight back under control!

You want to be happier again!

Be happier? Yes, this is also an extremely positive side effect of intermittent fasting, which you can often notice after 2 - 3 days of intermittent fasting.

Regular fasting increases your serotonin metabolism. And serotonin is known to be the human happiness hormone.

You'll be lucky if you notice that your scale shows less!

You are happy because you really manage to fast successfully, to stick to the intervals!

You are suddenly happy because you realize that through your self-discipline, you can no longer succumb to the temptation of quickly reaching for this or that "really delicious" calorie bomb as a snack. In short, your mood is stabilizing.

What will be interesting to pursue in the coming years are new scientific approaches that prove that regular fasting can also contribute to combating and preventing various neuronal diseases (e.g. Alzheimer's, ...).

Fatty Liver

Favored by the abundant and constantly available supply of food in our time and the often also existing lack of exercise, more and more people are overweight.
As a result, at some point the metabolism no longer functions properly and diseases such as cardiovascular diseases and diabetes develop. Intermittent fasting can help the metabolism to find its way back into balance.

The protein GADD45ß (Growth Arrest or DN Damage- inducible = THEN damage can be deduced) was investigated by a research team in Munich. This protein is linked to the cell cycle, repairs genetic damage and is also involved in the regulation of metabolism.

Tests on mice showed that the animals lacking GAAD45ß got fatty liver much faster because it controls fatty acid uptake in the liver.

Once the protein was restored, the fat content of the liver normalized, and the sugar metabolism improved.

In humans it could also be confirmed: the lower the GAAD45ß value, the higher the fat accumulation in the liver and the higher the blood sugar level.

Fasting means stress for the cells of the liver. This stress then stimulates the liver to produce more GAAD45ß and the body adapts to the new reduced food intake.

To bring the metabolism back into balance through intermittent fasting is therefore much more sensible and sustainable than taking medication.

If a fatty liver is avoided, this in turn has an influence on cardiovascular diseases, insulin resistance and possibly also on the growth of cancer cells.

Fibromyalgia

Fibromyalgia can also be described as fiber muscle pain.

It is a chronic condition of pain in muscle and tendon insertions, the cause of which is still unknown today. Fibromyalgia has a variety of symptoms, which for this reason often lead to false diagnoses. A distinction between rheumatism and other infectious diseases (Lyme disease) is also important, as the symptoms of these diseases are very similar.

The various accompanying symptoms of fibromyalgia are headaches, sleep disorders, exhaustion, nervousness, leg cramps and depressive moods.

In therapy, sports, physiotherapy, relaxation techniques and antidepressants are used above all. Alternatively, interval fasting is a good supplement. Because fasting reduces pain.

In a study conducted between 2005 and 2013, fibromyalgia patients with very different disease progressions were able to demonstrate a rapid reduction in pain and, in some cases, complete freedom from symptoms.

Unfortunately, apart from the results of this study, there is no special research that proves the connection between intermittent fasting and a cure for fibromyalgia.

However, intermittent fasting does not harm fibromyalgia patients under any circumstances and may provide relief after many years of chronic pain.

Detoxification and regeneration of the body

Mainly due to the oversupply of food, we eat too much and too frequently today. This food beyond the actual basic need impairs the natural renewal and cleansing process in our bodies.

The market has responded with special purification and detoxification products. Only the intake of those are of no use at all, if the way of food intake is not changed in a sustainable way.

As the history of fasting shows, humans are not naturally designed to require a permanent supply of food.

A constant change of food intake and hunger phases is much more effective for the metabolism.

Hormones and other substances such as adrenalin, HGH, glucagon, etc. stimulate and activate hunger.

In principle, the body signals: move, become active and go in search of food.

The body begins to draw on its fat reserves for energy production.

Digestion rests while fat burning is fully active.

The protein Sirtuine is only released in the state of hunger and checks and repairs all body cells (including DNA).

Whenever the body just starts to initiate this process, we eat something again and so purification and detoxification can never really get going.

An ideal model for detoxification and purification of the body is 16:8.

The body has 16 hours to initiate and carry out the regeneration and purification process undisturbed. The intestines are also cleaned.

The food taken in the time window of 8 hours is then much better absorbed and utilized by the body.

Further Advantages

➢ you give your body time to recover
➢ your sleep will get better
➢ you are less tired
➢ your metabolism is stimulated and increased again
➢ your immune system is strengthened
➢ hunger attacks become fewer and even disappear completely
➢ your body cells begin to purify themselves (autophagy)
➢ in the phases in which your pancreas does not release insulin, your cells are purified and repaired
➢ even skin aging is stopped (activation of anti-aging genes)

- by reducing the LDL value and increasing the HDL, the cholesterol level is optimized.
- also, the blood lipids are optimized
- too high blood pressure id returning to normal range
- weight loss not through loss of water or muscle mass, but through reduction of body fat
- weight reduction can prevent the onset of diabetes
- there is a very good chance that existing diabetes can be reversed
- inflammation in the body heals faster and better
- by the regeneration of the cells and the positively changed fat metabolism, it is also possible with a thyroid hypofunction to lose weight
- Cancer cells can be repaired
- the onset of cancer can be prevented
- can be easily integrated into everyday life
- you don't need "special foods," like many other "diets."

Drawbacks

Disadvantages of interval fasting are not known in healthy people.

Every now and then side effects are reported (individually different)

- ➢ Fatigue
    - o this often depends on your personal nutrition plan
    - o it usually appears in the evening
    - o take it as an opportunity to go to sleep early.
- ➢ Hunger
    - o permanent hunger is only a phenomenon of the adaptation period
    - o as soon as the metabolism has become accustomed, the hunger attacks also disappear
    - o your body learns relatively quickly to fall back on its sufficiently available reserves
- ➢ Unhealthy Nutrition = Danger

- often you can read that you can freely choose your foods during interval fasting
- but an unhealthy and unbalanced diet - especially at the beginning of intermittent fasting - can cause side effects:
  - headaches
  - halitosis
  - sickness
- There are people who experience fasting/long-term fasting as enormous stress

Tip:

If you start with intermittent fasting, it is a good time to consciously pay attention to your diet.

Avoid finished products, cook with fresh and natural foods, avoid sugar.

Also, intermittent fasting is not suitable for everyone, because there are a few limitations.

Intermittent fasting should be avoided when

- you are diabetic

- ➢ you are underweight
- ➢ if you are pregnant
- ➢ during lactation
- ➢ if it applies to you: without breakfast it doesn't work
- ➢ if you have known metabolic problems
- ➢ if you're suffering from hormone imbalances
- ➢ if you're suffering from blood sugar swings

If you're diabetic, it doesn't mean that right away intermittent fasting is not suitable for you!

No matter if you are diabetic or if you have been diagnosed with another disease: if you wish to give intermittent fasting a place in your life, please consult a doctor.

According to your individual state of health you can discuss the possibilities of intermittent fasting with your doctor!

What is important to note that intermittent fasting is successful?

Intermittent fasting requires self-discipline and the will to get through this time, especially in the initial phase, i.e. the changeover phase.

A few tips and suggestions can certainly help you:

- ➤ best start with small intervals - slowly approach and get the body used to fasting phases
- ➤ if possible, maintain the normal daily routine
- ➤ for the head: a failed meal is "eaten" via the body's own fat reserves
- ➤ follow the simple rules of the individual models and intermittent fasting in general
- ➤ a generally healthy and balanced diet is important
- ➤ be aware of the rules of your fasting model in advance (write them down until you have fully internalized them)
- ➤ if the first chosen method doesn't work properly (doesn't fit into your own schedule as expected

or is too hard to keep up), then try another model
- ➢ don't give up too fast: everybody gets used to fasting phases at different speeds!

Always keep in mind: intermittent fasting is the voluntary renunciation of food for a certain time or rhythm. You have chosen this one and yes, in the changeover phase you can get hungry.

Don't let the feeling of hunger become the dominant feeling, because you know when you take your next meal. If necessary, you can also take a healthy snack from the snack list.

But please only in the food window! So, all the positive change processes in your body can do their work undisturbed.

Risks

There are hardly any risks for a healthy person during intermittent fasting.

At least there are no meaningful medical studies on the subject yet.

Since intermittent fasting is a short and continuous fasting phase and you eat a healthy and balanced diet during the eating phases, your body will continue to be supplied with all the nutrients it needs to survive.

Many of the so-called miracle diets deny the body this or that group of nutrients.

Here, deficiency symptoms can easily develop and the danger of a "hunger metabolism" is extremely high.

But please always note: if you are diagnosed with a disease, if you take medication daily or if you already have diabetes, ... please first consult your doctor and discuss your plans with him!

The metabolism reacts quite differently during fasting.

Your normal dosage of medication may suddenly be too high during intermittent fasting and side effects or health complications may occur.

Here are mainly drugs such as beta blockers (lower blood pressure), blood thinners, (ASS, aspirin, ...), drainage tablets, antibiotics, cortisone, painkillers and rheumatism drugs.

Taking medication on an empty stomach is always a risk, but especially during fasting it is important to take the necessary medication after eating with plenty of water.

A good alternative for sedatives and painkillers is especially in intermittent fasting e.g. homeopathic remedies.

The use of homeopathic remedies for therapeutic purposes should also be discussed with a doctor.

If the doctor is of the opinion that the dose of medication must be reduced during intermittent fasting, it is absolutely necessary never to do this alone and arbitrarily.

Is it possible to make mistakes when fasting at intervals?

Yes, if you don't go into the intermittent fasting, the recommended dietary advice, etc. in detail beforehand, you can make mistakes:

> ➤ You can drink tea all day, but **never** make tea with honey.

- ➤ Honey destroys any fasting effect
- ➤ But there are other drinks that you should **not drink during** the fasting phase of your chosen model:
  - o Coffee with milk or coffee with sugar
  - o Espresso with sugar
  - o fruit juice
- ➤ **Ideal drinks:**
  - o to start the day: warm water with lemon
  - o ginger tea
  - o green tea
  - o black tea
  - o coffee/espresso
  - o water
  - o matcha tea
  - o Bulletproof Coffee

Good preparation is very important to avoid falling into error traps:

- ➤ plan for a week! It gives you something "to hold on to" by which you can orient yourself, for example when a hunger attack attacks your will and your self-discipline.

➢ make sure that you eat a healthy diet (rich in fibre and protein)

➢ if you want to take it seriously: remove all unhealthy food from your larder and fridge as a preparation.

   o so, you can't jump on the tempting treats during a ravenous hunger attack and ruin your previous successes.

   o replace your sugar supply with xylitol, stevia or birch sugar.

➢ in the meal window, you should eat enough, fill your stomach.

➢ if you feel an extreme feeling of hunger (do not confuse with appetite ☐), then you have taken too few calories.

➢ Coffee is allowed, but be careful anyway:

   o If you drink black coffee in the morning on an empty stomach, your body reacts more strongly than during the day.

      ▪ it produces adrenaline

- more insulin is released as a result
  - **Tip:** start your day with a Bulletproof Coffee
- don't change your mealtimes from day to day.
  - keep the interval between meals as your body will enjoy this regularity.
- wrong and too heavy food makes you tired.
- if dinner is very carbohydrate heavy, or if you treat yourself to something sweet in the evening, you may feel more hungry than usual the next morning

(release of more blood sugar in the evening)

Types of Intermittent Fasting

Hours Fasting

Intermittent fasting is hours of fasting since you are always fasting for a predetermined number of hours. This hour of fasting/intermittent fasting is a planned and controlled fasting with always the same basic conditions.

By this kind of fasting, the conscious decision for a fasting model and the basic conditions, the psychological and mental stress, which arises with a hunger attack, can be avoided.

During the changeover there will be hunger attacks, but you know immediately that you can eat again soon or drink tea/coffee immediately.

Hunger Fasting

Fasting is the voluntary renunciation of food for a certain period of time or, as with intermittent fasting, in a certain rhythm.

Hunger arises from a wide variety of causes, is usually unwanted and becomes a dominant feeling.

If hunger cannot be satisfied, this leads to a lack of appetite, changes in the central nervous system and then to stress reactions.

Since intermittent fasting is a conscious, voluntary and deliberate action, there are no fear or stress reactions.

All the positive change processes in the body can do their work undisturbed.

Models of Intermittent Fasting

<u>**1:6**</u>

1 day (24 hours) fasting

6 days normal, health-conscious nutrition

On 6 days a week you can eat healthy and balanced and on one day (24 hours) you fast.

During your fasting day you will only drink enough liquids (tea, homemade vegetable juices, mineral water).

If you fast "only" 1 day a week, you will have it a little easier, because e.g. constantly recurring hunger attacks (mostly however only in the phase of the change) are not superficial

This 1 day fasting/week is not suitable to lose much weight but is good for the body.

During the remaining 6 days, eat a healthy and balanced diet.

The day following the fasting day should, if possible, be your "protein day". For this day consciously choose protein-rich foods. This increases the effect of the fasting day a little.

2:5

2 days/week fasting

5 days/week normal, health-conscious diet

5 days a week you eat a healthy and balanced diet and on the remaining 2 days the calorie intake is reduced to a minimum.

The guideline values here are approx. 500 kcal for women and approx. 600 kcal for men.

It is important not to place the two calorie-reduced days directly behind each other. You have the possibility to choose the 2 days/week that make the most sense for you and fit best into your weekly schedule.

1:1

1 day (24 hours) fasting

1 day (24 hours) normal, health-conscious diet

You can certainly try out this model as an increase after a successful familiarization with the 5:2 rhythm. 1 day (24 hours) you eat normally and healthy and on the following day (24 hours) you adhere to the calorie-reduced rule of 5: 2 fasting (women = 500 kcal and men = 600 kcal).

As soon as you get used to this rhythm, you can gradually reduce or omit the calorie-reduced food and only take calorie-free drinks, possibly a broth.

Important: this method is not suitable for people with health problems or for beginners.
You need a very high degree of self-discipline!

16/8

16 hours fasting
8-hour meal window (3 meals)

An increase of the 12 hours of fasting is the 16: 8 model.
You fast 16 hours and have an 8-hour window for your food intake.

In these 8 hours, however, only a maximum of three meals are allowed (in order to achieve the best effect). It is also ideal to combine this rhythm with your daily bedtime. A possible guideline, for example, would be to have the last meal at 7 p.m. in the evening and then have the first meal at 11 a.m. on the following day. Basically, you're skipping breakfast. That's why the 16:8 model is also quite suitable for you if you hardly ever have breakfast.
You can divide the 16:8 hours into the hours that best fit your individual daily schedule.

20/4
20 hours fasting

4-hour meal window

The 20-hour fasting method and a 4-hour food intake window is also called a "Warrior diet".

During the 4-hour window you can eat anything you like.
So that the 20-hour fasting phase does not become too long, a calorie intake of 500 kcal for women and 600 kcal for men is permitted here as with 1: 1 fasting.
Fruits, juices and vegetables are the most suitable.

36/12
36 hours fasting
12-hour meal window

Fasting in 36:12 is a great challenge and only suitable for very few people.
Food intake takes place within 12 hours (exactly defined from 8 a.m. to 8 p.m.).

Then there's a 36-hour meal break till the morning after tomorrow.

During this break, a sufficient supply of fluids is very important! On the morning after tomorrow at 8 am food can be gutted again.

This is how intermittent fasting works!

Since every person is different, there is also no right or wrong entry into the intermittent fasting.

There are people who approach the intermittent fasting in steps.

Others can enter the fasting interval from one day to the next in their chosen model.

Here are a few tips and tricks to help you get started with intermittent fasting:

> ➢ if you generally eat 4 or 5 meals (incl. snacks) a day, reduce this to breakfast, lunch and dinner (cancel all snacks)

- as soon as you feel comfortable with 3 meals a day, you can start taking breakfast later and later
- maybe you'll find out that you don't really need breakfast any more at some point
- ideally the breakfast consists of raw vegetables, smoothies, salad, ...
- for lunch, for example, healthy fats are ideal
- In the evening you can eat whatever you want
- important: shift the times of your meals as you feel good with them
- you will feel it when you can consciously step into your chosen model
- ideal is the 16: 8 model, because it is the most adapted to our daily rhythm

Remember: you have consciously decided to integrate intermittent fasting into your life.

In the phases when a hunger attack attacks you, look at the clock, perhaps there are only 60 minutes left until the next meal. Stay strong, distract yourself, chew sugar-free gum, or drink warm tea or coffee.

If you don't make it now, getting used to and changing will be much more difficult, even impossible for some people, because they quickly fall back into old eating patterns.

If you hold on, not only will your self-confidence increase (I have passed the first hurdle), but you will also feel the first positive changes (through already started detoxification and purification).

After getting used to 3 meals a day, your day could look like this in the 16:8 model:

- ➤ your last day of "normal" dinner ends in the evening with a dinner of your choice. Make sure you finish dinner at 7:00.
- ➤ after 7:00, until you go to sleep, you can still drink tea, water or coffee.
- ➤ **11:00** and it's time for your breakfast. A protein-rich breakfast is recommended:
  - o Bacon, fried egg, baked beans

If you'd rather have a carbohydrate-rich breakfast:
  - o bread rolls, jam (best sugar - reduced)

- ➤ Ginger tea acts as a fat booster (can be drunk all day), but also any other tea and coffee for breakfast is allowed
- ➤ a saturating shake for breakfast is a healthy and tasty alternative
- ➤ **3:00 p.m.** and you can have a healthy and satisfying lunch.
  - ○ Chicken breast with noodles or rice

Eating full is important here. If you like, you can have a piece of cake for dessert

- ➤ **Sport** would be a good thing before the last meal of the day
- ➤ if the hunger is particularly noticeable now, you can eat some fruit or vegetables as a snack. A few nuts or almonds are good too. If the longing for chocolate is great, you can also enjoy a few pieces of dark chocolate with 85 % cocoa.
- ➤ **7 p.m.**

Since you should be ready with dinner at 7 p.m., it is important that you start the preparation in time. Assume you need 15 minutes to eat yourself.

- ➢ although you have a free choice of dinner, it would be a good idea to choose a low carb dish in the evening. One reason for this is that you won't get an insulin peak (hunger attack) for the rest of the evening.
- ➢ from **7 p.m. to 11 a.m. on the following day,** your fasting phase begins.
- ➢ in the evening and throughout the day, it is important that you drink enough and also pay attention to your choice of drinks:
    - ○ Water
    - ○ ginger tea
    - ○ green tea
    - ○ black tea
    - ○ coffee - but without milk and/or sugar

Depending on how your day goes, you can of course adapt the mealtimes to your daily routine.

You can also put your fasting phase of 16 hours like this:

- ➢ 6 p.m. to 10 a.m.
- ➢ 20 o'clock to 12 o'clock

➤ 9 p.m. to 1 p.m.

➤ 5 p.m. to 9 a.m.

➤ ...

If you work the shift system or always only work the night shift, you plan your meals during your working hours and the fasting phase into your bedtime.

The 16: 8 model of intermittent fasting is a very flexible one.

Tips and Tricks:

➤ avoid a negative calorie balance = it is important that you cover at least your daily calories basic requirement, because otherwise your body comes fast into a deficit

➤ Avoid Binge-Eating (BES) or "eating attacks", especially in the evening or after the fasting phase

➤ distribute your calories evenly throughout the day and do this consciously right from the start of the changeover. So, you not only get used to the rhythm of time, but also to your food portions at the same time

- continue to participate in your social life. Even a visit to a restaurant in the evening is not a problem, except perhaps time (keeping the time window is important)
- if you experience hunger attacks inside the food window, the best way to fight them is with a warm drink, a healthy snack from the list, or by chewing sugar-free chewing gum
- you can only counter hunger attacks in the fasting window with a warm drink
- sleep sufficiently, because while you sleep you do not feel hungry and at the same time your body and mind recover and you have enough energy and willpower for the new day again.
- don't try to "catch up" on cancelled meals
- your own willpower is very much in demand, especially in the first weeks, because your body does not always accept such a change simply like that
- always make yourself aware: a failed meal is supplemented from your "fat depot"

- ➢ just in the beginning: please do not force your own body to something by bending and breaking
- ➢ the diet should be generally healthy and balanced:
  - o rich in dietary fibre and protein:
  - o vegetables
  - o lean meat
  - o fish
  - o oat flakes
  - o Quinoa, Bulgur
  - o ....

- ➢ <u>Good snacks in the range of 500 kcal/woman and 600 kcal/man are for example:</u>
  - o 100 gr. blueberries (approx. 60 kcal)
  - o 100 gr. apricots (approx. 43 kcal)
  - o 100 gr. apple (ca.52 kcal)
  - o 100 gr. strawberries (approx. 32 kcal)
  - o 100 gr. cauliflower (approx. 25 kcal)
  - o 100 gr. broccoli (approx. 35 kcal)
  - o 100 gr. cucumber (approx. 15 kcal)

- o 100gr. carrot (approx. 36 kcal)
- o 100gr. chicken breast (approx. 75 kcal)
- o 100 gr. veal (approx. 94 kcal)
- o 100 gr. beef (approx. 115 Kcal)
- o 100 gr. saithe fillet (approx. 83 kcal)
- o 100 gr. tuna (approx. 144 kcal)
- o 100 gr. buttermilk (approx. 38 kcal)
- o 100 gr. milk (approx. 47 kcal)
- o 100 gr. natural yoghurt (approx. 62 kcal)
- o 100gr. ribbon noodles cooked (approx. 142 kcal)
- o 100 gr. spelt noodles cooked (approx. 128 kcal)
- o 1 hard-boiled egg (approx. 75 Kcal)
- o 1 tablespoon humus (approx. 53 kcal)
- o 1 cup miso soup (approx. 32 kcal)

So there are a lot of snacks that are healthy and are available to a balanced diet as a snack during the long fasting phases.

How long can I use Intermittent Fasting?

As already mentioned above, the intermittent fasting is not a diet, but a lifestyle.

If the period of acclimatization is over, the rhythm you choose is very quickly your life.

You automatically stick to your time windows; you also eat more consciously and healthier.

If, after a short time, the positive effects, such as weight loss, less fatigue, balance, an all-round better body feeling, ... are added, you don't want to live any other way.

There is no time limit for intermittent fasting!

Nevertheless, a few aspects are still pointed out at this point:

Especially in the beginning, when your body is getting used to the other rhythm, it can sometimes come to exhaustion and the feeling of being permanently hungry.

However, this is usually only of short duration.

Holding out is important now.

Your body gets used to the new quite quickly and the hunger is covered by the body reserves.

In the beginning time it can happen that you are tired early in the evening. Just take this as an opportunity to go to sleep early.

Slight nausea, bad breath and headaches have also been observed as initial side effects.

Usually, however, they disappear again after a short time.

Caution is advised, however, if there is a pre-existing condition such as depression, if you are permanently exposed to an increased level of stress or if you are pregnant:

Intermittent fasting can be rather harmful here, since the body must be constantly supplied with nutrients.

If you have eating disorders (sugar addiction, ...) or depression, you should not start fasting at intervals alone.

If it is absolutely desired or if it is necessary for medical reasons, then it would be a good idea to initiate and supervise the changeover on an inpatient basis.

Can interval fasting be addictive?

It is well known that we like to use carbohydrates and fats (sweets, snacks, ... in excess) during periods of strong emotional stress, fear, excessive sadness, ...

This can quickly lead to an addiction in "susceptible" people.

The question of whether intermittent fasting can be addictive is therefore not quite so far-fetched.

These "vulnerable" people can discover the psychological effects of intermittent fasting as a new way to cope with their fears, stress, sadness, ...

Through the mood-stabilizing effects of intermittent fasting, it could happen that these people get into a kind of vicious circle.

They are then anxious to stay in this state of hunger as long as possible and do not manage to break the vicious circle without help.

It can happen that the health-promoting intermittent fasting is used as an introduction to a massive eating disorder (anorexia, bulimia, ...).

Studies on Intermittent Fasting

As already mentioned, there are virtually no scientifically based studies on intermittent fasting. In the area of sport, however, there are studies that deal with intermittent fasting and sport.

There are high-performance athletes (marathon runners, strength athletes, ...) who even report that their ability to concentrate was increased and their body fat percentage reduced while they were still fasting.

The sleep behavior itself was also perceived as significantly better, which improved the overall well-being and increased performance.

A study with competitive athletes was summarized as follows:

"These results show that the blood sugar level in humans remains at a normal level during training, even after a fasting phase and this despite the empty liver glycogen storage."

The body of an athlete gets its energy from the fat cells and this leads to an increased fat burning and fat mobilization.

The level of growth hormones also rises during the fasting hours.

For women this was on average 1,300 %, for men even 2,000 %.

In 2016, a study on intermittent fasting among strength athletes came to the conclusion that strength athletes who practiced 16:8 intermittent fasting (3 meals at 1 pm, 4 pm and 8 pm) lost an average of 1.6 kg of body fat. A comparison group that did not fast at the same time and consumed the same number of calories with 3 meals (1 pm, 4 pm and 8 pm) could not show any reduction in body fat.

Muscle mass and strength remained the same in both groups.

A 2018 study (Journal of the International Society of Sports) selected a model of 4: 3.

4 days/week the athletes consumed 2.350 kcal/day, and 3 days 1.300 kcal/day.

After 6 weeks, tests were performed that were amazing:

➢ 15 % less body fat
➢ 3 % more muscle mass
➢ improved lactate levels
➢ lower heart rate (for the same workout)
➢ less fatigue
➢ generally improved performance
➢ faster regeneration capacity

In another study, the subjects fasted for 3.5 days. Only then was their athletic performance measured using various parameters. Almost all values were not affected by the intermittent fasting. Only the isokinetic force of the muscle was reduced by about 10 %.

2 forces work in the muscle during sporting activity:

- isokinetic force (under movement, force that the muscle applies when, for example, pulling a weight towards itself or pushing it away)
- isometric force (static force, force used to hold a weight, for example)

However, it is assumed that the loss of 10% of isokinetic force is due to the 3.5 day fasting period prior to the study. During a normal fasting rhythm in the course of the intermittent fasting such a loss of strength is not assumed.

It seems to be optimal to exercise in a sober state (e.g. after the 16-hour fasting period).

It does not matter whether it is endurance or strength training.

After sport the eating period can be started normally.

Intermittent Fasting - the oldest form of fasting in modern times

Intermittent fasting is not witchcraft.

The most important thing is to find the model that is best for you to implement, the best to integrate into your normal everyday life.

If there are any signs of a disease or if such a disease has already been diagnosed (diabetes, ...), please discuss in advance with your doctor whether intermittent fasting is possible for you, and if so, which model is best for you!

Intermittent fasting is - especially in the beginning - a matter of attitude: your self-discipline, your willpower and your stamina are required (sudden hunger attacks, ...)!

Please ALWAYS make sure that there is a sufficient supply of liquid!

Unsweetened tea and/or coffee, water, water, water!

During long fasting phases / fasting days (5: 2, 24 hours fasting, ...) a limited calorie intake (women 500 kcal / men 600 kcal) is allowed and important.

Here, just at noon, besides the whole snack alternatives, a vegetable or chicken soup is offered. It fills your stomach sustainably.

A warm, sugar-free drink in between is also a good remedy against ravenous hunger attacks.

Make sure that the portion size of your individual meals is not larger than before!

Keep your portion sizes, but now maybe with the better, healthier foods:

Vegetables (= fibre), dairy products, eggs, fish, meat, pulses, mushrooms, nuts (= protein sources).

If your chosen model provides 2 meals during the eating phase, stick to it!

Avoid snacks! But if there is no other way, then choose them consciously (see list above)!

If you have decided on the 5:2 model, plan your fasting days so that they are relatively quiet days for you. And never fast two days in a row!

Plan your meals! Especially at the beginning it can be important and helpful if you write down a meal plan. Plan a week in advance what you want to eat and when.

Buy all required ingredients beforehand, so that you already have them at home.

There are many recipes on the Internet that are specially designed for intermittent fasting.

Here you will surely find something you like.

You are also always free to vary a little within the recipes with the ingredients.

For example, if you don't like figs, you can use a plum or apricot instead.

If you don't like chili, maybe wasabi is an alternative that you like.

Choose the healthy ingredients so that your food is delicious and tasty for you.

Don't be shy, experiment with the "allowed" foods (the good and right ones ☐).

Regular exercise is also important.

Because little movement gives your body the signal "shortage " and it grabs every available calorie and stores it.

Sleep! Yes, with 7 - 8 hours of sleep you have a much better starting point to reach your goal and it is easier for you to survive the day.

And then there's the stress. Stress sneaks far too often into all the different areas of your life!

If you have too much stress (whether physical or psychological) your body produces more cortisol. And this nice hormone causes an increased storage of the absorbed energy in fat deposits in your body.

Intermittent fasting does not need a "Cheat Day" like many other diets.

Let's do it!

You can start intermittent fasting every day!

Prepare yourself well!

Choose the model that suits you best!

Follow the respective rules!

In case of doubt, talk to a doctor first!

Hang in there if hunger catches you cold in the beginning!

It is worth it, because you will soon feel the positive changes in your body!

Incorporate your form of intermittent fasting into your life so that it feels good.

This way you can guarantee that the changeover will be successful, and that intermittent fasting will soon be a normal part of your daily routine.

Disclaimer

The implementation of all information, instructions and strategies contained in this book is at your own risk. The author cannot assume any liability for any damages of any kind for any legal reason. Liability claims regarding damage caused by the use of any information provided, including any kind of information which is incomplete or incorrect, will therefore be rejected. Any legal claims and claims for damages are therefore also excluded. This work has been written down with the greatest care to the best of our knowledge and belief. For the topicality, completeness and quality of the information the author takes over however no guarantee. Printing errors and false information can also not be completely excluded. No legal responsibility or liability in any form can be assumed for incorrect information provided by the author.

Copyright

www.ingramcontent.com/pod-product-compliance
Lightning Source LLC
Chambersburg PA
CBHW020329290526
45785CB00007B/2972